Dietary Restrictions and Allergies

Your Guide to Living Well with Dietary Challenges

Labanya Tandi

Copyright Page

Dietary Restrictions and Allergies

Disclaimer: The information provided in this ebook is intended for general knowledge and informational purposes only, and does not constitute medical advice. Readers should consult with a healthcare professional for any medical concerns or before making any significant changes to their diet or lifestyle.

contact @ Blazebeefofficial@gmail.com

Table of Contents

Dedication... 3

Table of Contents 4

Acknowledgments 6

Introduction... 7

The Epidemic of Dietary Restrictions and Allergies 7

The Challenges Faced by Individuals with Dietary Restrictions and Allergies 9

The Importance of Understanding and Accommodating Dietary Needs................................. 10

Chapter 1 : Understanding Dietary Restrictions and Allergies 12

Common Dietary Restrictions... 12

Common Food Allergies... 13

Allergies vs. Intolerances... 14

The Impact of Dietary Restrictions and Allergies on Physical and Mental Health................. 15

Chapter 2 : Navigating the Food Environment... 17

Reading Food Labels and Understanding Ingredient Lists.. 17

Finding Safe and Enjoyable Dining Options 18

Eating Out with Dietary Restrictions.. 19

Traveling with Food Allergies.. 20

Cooking at Home with Dietary Considerations 21

Chapter 3 : Creating a Nutritious Diet... 23

Building Balanced Meals with Dietary Restrictions.. 23

Finding Alternative Sources of Nutrients 25

Meal Planning and Preparation Tips.. 26

The Role of Supplements.. 28

Addressing Common Nutritional Concerns... 30

Chapter 4 : Overcoming Challenges **32**

Coping with Social and Emotional Aspects of Dietary Restrictions 32

Communicating Dietary Needs Effectively 34

Building a Support Network 35

Finding Online Resources and Communities 37

Chapter 5 : Specific Dietary Restrictions and Allergies **39**

In-Depth Information on Specific Dietary Conditions 39

Common Allergies 40

Conclusion **41**

take control of your dietary health 41

The future of food is inclusive and exciting. 42

About the Author **43**

Acknowledgments

I would like to express my sincere gratitude to Bhuban. His support and encouragement was invaluable in bringing this book to fruition.

I am also grateful Blazebeef for providing valuable resources and information.

Lastly, I would like to thank my readers for their interest in this topic. Your support means the world to me.

Introduction

The Epidemic of Dietary Restrictions and Allergies

The landscape of food consumption has undergone a dramatic transformation in recent decades. Once a matter of personal preference or cultural tradition, dietary restrictions and food allergies have evolved into a pervasive public health concern. The implications of this shift are far-reaching, affecting individuals, healthcare systems, and the food industry alike.

Historically, food sensitivities were often isolated incidents, with limited societal impact. However, a confluence of factors has contributed to the exponential growth of these conditions. Among the most significant is the heightened awareness of the connection between diet and health. As scientific research continues to illuminate the intricate relationship between food, the immune system, and chronic disease, individuals are increasingly scrutinizing their dietary choices. This heightened consciousness has led to a surge in the identification and management of food-related issues.

Environmental factors have also played a pivotal role in the escalation of dietary restrictions and allergies. The widespread use of pesticides, herbicides, and antibiotics in agriculture has altered the composition of our food supply. Additionally, the prevalence of processed foods, laden with additives and preservatives, has disrupted the delicate balance of the human gut microbiome. These environmental stressors have been implicated in the development of food sensitivities and autoimmune disorders.

The globalization of food systems has introduced a complex array of allergens into the diet. As consumers have access to a wider variety of foods from around the world, the potential for exposure to unfamiliar allergens has increased. Moreover, the prevalence of food additives and cross-contamination in food processing facilities has exacerbated the problem.

The rise of social media has amplified the discourse surrounding dietary restrictions and allergies. Online platforms have facilitated the sharing of personal experiences and information, fostering a sense of community among individuals with these conditions. While this has been beneficial in raising awareness, it has also contributed to the spread of misinformation and fear-mongering.

The consequences of this epidemic are multifaceted. Individuals with dietary restrictions and allergies often face significant challenges in navigating the food environment. Social isolation, limited food options, and the constant vigilance required to avoid triggers can have a profound impact on quality of life. Moreover, the economic burden associated with specialized diets and healthcare costs can be substantial.

The food industry has responded to this growing trend by introducing a wider range of allergy-friendly and specialized products. However, the challenge of ensuring food safety and accurately labeling products remains complex. The need for clear and comprehensive allergen information is paramount to protect consumers with food allergies.

Healthcare providers play a critical role in the management of dietary restrictions and allergies. Accurate diagnosis, education, and support are essential for individuals living with these conditions. As the prevalence of these conditions continues to rise, there is a growing need for specialized training and resources for healthcare professionals.

epidemic of dietary restrictions and allergies represents a significant public health challenge. Addressing this issue requires a multi-faceted approach involving individuals, healthcare providers, the food industry, and policymakers. By fostering a greater understanding of these conditions, promoting research, and implementing supportive policies, we can work towards a future where everyone can enjoy food without fear.

The Challenges Faced by Individuals with Dietary Restrictions and Allergies

Living with dietary restrictions or food allergies presents a unique set of challenges that profoundly impact daily life. These individuals must navigate a complex and often hostile food environment, while also managing the psychological and emotional toll of their conditions.

One of the most significant challenges is the constant vigilance required to avoid triggers. Individuals with food allergies must meticulously read food labels, inquire about ingredients in restaurants, and exercise caution when attending social events. This level of hypervigilance can be exhausting and isolating. Fear of accidental exposure to allergens, known as anaphylaxis, can lead to anxiety and a sense of restricted freedom.

Dietary restrictions also pose significant social challenges. Sharing meals with friends and family can become a source of stress and anxiety. The limited availability of suitable food options often leads to feelings of exclusion and social isolation. Dining out can be a daunting experience, as navigating menus and communicating dietary needs can be overwhelming.

The psychological impact of dietary restrictions and allergies cannot be overstated. The constant worry about food safety can lead to anxiety, depression, and low self-esteem. Children with these conditions may experience bullying or teasing from peers, further exacerbating their emotional distress. Moreover, the grief associated with the loss of favorite foods can be a significant challenge.

Beyond the emotional toll, individuals with dietary restrictions often face practical difficulties. Access to safe and nutritious food can be limited, especially in rural areas or for those with low incomes. The cost of specialized foods can be exorbitant, placing a financial burden on families. Additionally, traveling can be a stressful experience, as finding suitable food options while away from home can be challenging.

Individuals with dietary restrictions and allergies face a multitude of challenges that impact their physical, emotional, and social well-being. Addressing these challenges requires a comprehensive approach that involves education, support, and policy changes. By fostering a more inclusive and understanding society, we can help to improve the quality of life for those living with these conditions.

The Importance of Understanding and Accommodating Dietary Needs

Understanding and accommodating dietary needs is paramount to fostering a healthy, inclusive, and respectful environment. Whether in homes, schools, workplaces, or public spaces, recognizing and respecting diverse dietary requirements is essential for promoting well-being and preventing negative health outcomes.

For individuals with food allergies or intolerances, accommodating their needs is crucial to prevent severe allergic reactions and ensure their safety. Even trace amounts of allergens can be life-threatening, emphasizing the importance of careful food preparation and clear labeling. By understanding and respecting these dietary restrictions, we create a safe space for those with allergies to participate fully in social and communal activities.

Beyond safety, accommodating dietary needs is a matter of inclusivity and respect. Everyone deserves to feel valued and included, regardless of their dietary choices. By offering diverse food options and creating an environment where dietary restrictions are understood and honored, we promote a sense of belonging and acceptance.

Moreover, understanding dietary needs can contribute to overall health and well-being. Many dietary restrictions are based on health considerations, such as managing chronic diseases, maintaining a healthy weight, or following specific medical advice. By accommodating these needs, we support individuals in achieving their health goals.

In the realm of hospitality and food service, understanding and accommodating dietary needs is essential for customer satisfaction. Offering a variety of options, including vegetarian, vegan, gluten-free, and allergen-free choices, demonstrates a commitment to meeting the needs of a diverse clientele.

In conclusion, understanding and accommodating dietary needs is a fundamental aspect of creating a healthy, inclusive, and respectful society. By prioritizing the needs of individuals with dietary restrictions, we promote safety, well-being, and a sense of belonging.

Chapter 1 : Understanding Dietary Restrictions and Allergies

Common Dietary Restrictions

Dietary restrictions encompass a wide range of food exclusions based on various factors, including health, ethics, and personal preference. Some of the most common dietary restrictions include vegetarianism, veganism, gluten-free, and dairy-free diets.

Vegetarianism involves abstaining from consuming meat, poultry, and seafood. However, the definition of vegetarianism can vary widely. Lacto-ovo vegetarians consume dairy products and eggs, while lacto vegetarians include only dairy products. Vegans, on the other hand, exclude all animal-derived products, including meat, poultry, fish, eggs, dairy, and honey. Their dietary choices are often motivated by ethical, environmental, or health concerns.

Gluten-free diets eliminate gluten, a protein found in wheat, barley, and rye. Celiac disease is an autoimmune condition that necessitates a gluten-free diet. However, many individuals choose to follow this diet for perceived health benefits or to manage gluten sensitivity.

Dairy-free diets exclude milk and milk products, including cheese, butter, yogurt, and ice cream. Lactose intolerance, a digestive disorder, is a common reason for adopting a dairy-free diet. However, some individuals choose to eliminate dairy for ethical or health reasons.

It's important to note that these are just a few examples of common dietary restrictions. Other restrictions may include nut-free, soy-free, or shellfish-free diets, often due to allergies or intolerances. Additionally, religious and cultural practices can influence dietary choices, leading to specific food exclusions.

Common Food Allergies

Food allergies are immune system responses to specific food proteins. While anyone can develop a food allergy at any age, certain foods are more commonly associated with allergic reactions.

Nuts are a frequent culprit in food allergies. This category includes tree nuts such as almonds, walnuts, cashews, and pecans, as well as peanuts, which are technically legumes. Reactions to nuts can range from mild to severe, with some individuals experiencing life-threatening anaphylaxis.

Shellfish is another common allergen. This category encompasses crustaceans like shrimp, crab, and lobster, as well as mollusks like clams, oysters, and mussels. Shellfish allergies often develop in adulthood and can persist throughout life.

Soy is a plant-based protein that can trigger allergic reactions in some individuals. Soy is found in a variety of products, including tofu, soy milk, and soy sauce, making it essential for those with soy allergies to carefully read food labels.

It's important to note that these are just a few examples of common food allergies. Other allergens include milk, eggs, wheat, fish, and sesame. While the severity of food allergies can vary widely, even mild reactions can significantly impact quality of life.

Allergies vs. Intolerances

While both allergies and intolerances involve adverse reactions to food, they are distinct conditions with different underlying mechanisms and symptoms.

Food allergies are immune system responses to specific food proteins. When a person with a food allergy consumes the allergen, their immune system mistakenly identifies it as a threat and releases chemicals, including histamine, to attack it. This can lead to a range of symptoms, from mild to severe, including hives, swelling, difficulty breathing, and in severe cases, anaphylaxis. Food allergies are often persistent and require strict avoidance of the offending food.

Food intolerances, on the other hand, do not involve the immune system. Instead, they result from the body's inability to properly digest or process certain food components. Common examples include lactose intolerance, where the body lacks the enzyme lactase to digest lactose, and gluten intolerance, where the body has difficulty digesting gluten. Symptoms of food intolerances are typically less severe than allergies and often involve digestive issues such as bloating, gas, diarrhea, and abdominal pain.

It's important to note that while food allergies and intolerances can share some overlapping symptoms, they require different management strategies. Allergic reactions can be life-threatening, necessitating strict avoidance of the allergen. Food intolerances may require dietary modifications or the use of digestive enzymes.

The Impact of Dietary Restrictions and Allergies on Physical and Mental Health

Dietary restrictions and allergies can significantly impact both physical and mental health. These conditions often necessitate substantial lifestyle adjustments, which can have far-reaching consequences.

Physical Health:

Nutritional deficiencies: Adhering to restrictive diets can make it challenging to consume a balanced range of nutrients. Deficiencies in essential vitamins, minerals, and macronutrients can lead to various health problems, including fatigue, weakened immune system, and impaired cognitive function.

Digestive issues: Many dietary restrictions are implemented to manage digestive problems. While eliminating certain foods may alleviate symptoms, it can also disrupt the gut microbiome, potentially leading to further digestive disturbances.

Allergic reactions: Food allergies pose a constant threat to physical health. Severe allergic reactions, such as anaphylaxis, can be life-threatening. Even mild reactions can cause discomfort, inflammation, and impaired daily functioning.

Mental Health:

Anxiety and stress: The constant vigilance required to avoid allergens or adhere to dietary restrictions can lead to chronic stress and anxiety. Fear of accidental exposure to allergens can significantly impact quality of life.

Social isolation: Dietary limitations can create challenges in social settings, as food often plays a central role in social interactions. This can lead to feelings of isolation and loneliness.

Body image and self-esteem: Restrictive diets can contribute to disordered eating patterns and negative body image. The constant focus on food and dietary rules can negatively impact self-esteem.

Depression: The cumulative effects of physical symptoms, social challenges, and emotional distress associated with dietary restrictions and allergies can increase the risk of depression.

It's important to note that the impact of dietary restrictions and allergies varies widely among individuals. While some people manage these challenges effectively, others may experience more significant physical and mental health consequences.

Chapter 2 : Navigating the Food Environment

Reading Food Labels and Understanding Ingredient Lists

Reading food labels and understanding ingredient lists is essential for making informed dietary choices. This skill is particularly crucial for individuals with dietary restrictions, allergies, or specific health goals.

Food labels provide valuable information about a product's nutritional content, serving size, and ingredients. The ingredient list is typically found on the back or side of the package and displays all components used in the product, listed in descending order by weight. The first ingredient is the most abundant, followed by the next most abundant, and so on.

Understanding common food additives and processing terms is crucial for interpreting ingredient lists. Hidden sources of allergens, unhealthy fats, excessive sugars, or artificial sweeteners can be identified by carefully examining the ingredients.

For individuals with dietary restrictions, reading food labels is vital to avoid prohibited ingredients. Those with allergies must meticulously check for potential allergens, often hidden under different names. Similarly, people following specific diets, such as low-sodium, low-sugar, or gluten-free, need to scrutinize the label to ensure the product aligns with their dietary goals.

While food labels offer essential information, it's important to be aware of their limitations. Serving sizes can be misleading, and some labels may use marketing claims that can be deceptive. Therefore, relying solely on food labels without considering other factors, such as the overall nutritional quality of the product, is not recommended.

By developing the ability to read and understand food labels, individuals can make more informed choices about the foods they consume and improve their overall health and well-being.

Finding Safe and Enjoyable Dining Options

Dining out can be a social and enjoyable experience, but it presents unique challenges for individuals with dietary restrictions or allergies. Finding safe and satisfying food options requires careful planning and effective communication.

One of the primary challenges is identifying restaurants that can accommodate specific dietary needs. Researching establishments beforehand can be time-consuming, but it's often worth the effort. Many restaurants now offer online menus or allergen information, which can be helpful in making informed decisions.

Effective communication with restaurant staff is essential. Clearly and concisely explaining dietary restrictions is crucial to avoid misunderstandings. It's helpful to be prepared to provide detailed information about allergens or ingredients to avoid. Some individuals find it beneficial to carry a card or document outlining their dietary needs.

While finding safe options is important, it's equally essential to discover enjoyable dining experiences. Exploring different cuisines and trying new dishes can be a rewarding part of the dining process. Many restaurants offer a variety of dishes that can be adapted to accommodate dietary restrictions. Additionally, seeking out restaurants that specialize in specific cuisines or dietary preferences can increase the likelihood of finding satisfying options.

Ultimately, finding safe and enjoyable dining options requires patience, persistence, and a willingness to explore different establishments. With careful planning and effective communication, individuals with dietary restrictions can discover delicious and satisfying dining experiences.

Eating Out with Dietary Restrictions

Eating out with dietary restrictions can be a challenging experience, but with careful planning and effective communication, it is possible to enjoy a satisfying meal.

One of the biggest challenges is navigating restaurant menus, which can be overwhelming for those with specific dietary needs. Deciphering ingredients, identifying potential cross-contamination risks, and finding suitable options can be time-consuming and stressful. Many individuals with dietary restrictions rely on restaurant staff to provide accurate information and accommodate their needs.

Effective communication is essential when dining out. Clearly and concisely explaining dietary restrictions to the server is crucial to avoid misunderstandings. It is often helpful to provide a written list of allergens or dietary requirements to ensure accurate order placement. Additionally, asking questions about preparation methods and ingredients can help to minimize the risk of unintended exposure to problematic foods.

Social dynamics can also play a role in the dining out experience for individuals with dietary restrictions. Feeling excluded or pressured to compromise their dietary needs can be emotionally challenging. It is important to establish open and honest communication with dining companions to ensure everyone feels comfortable and supported.

While dining out can present obstacles, it is important to remember that many restaurants are becoming increasingly accommodating to diverse dietary needs. By being prepared, communicating effectively, and maintaining a positive attitude, individuals with dietary restrictions can enjoy a pleasurable dining experience.

Traveling with Food Allergies

Traveling with food allergies can be a daunting task, requiring careful planning and preparation. Navigating unfamiliar environments, language barriers, and different culinary practices can pose significant challenges.

One of the primary concerns is ensuring access to necessary medications. Carrying an adequate supply of allergy medication, including epinephrine auto-injectors, is crucial. It's essential to pack these items in carry-on luggage to avoid losing them during checked baggage handling. Additionally, it's advisable to inform airline personnel about the allergy and carry a doctor's note if necessary.

Researching the destination is key to managing food allergies effectively. Understanding local cuisine, common allergens in the region, and the availability of allergen-free options can help in planning meals and avoiding potential risks. Learning basic phrases related to food allergies in the local language can facilitate communication with restaurant staff.

Packing safe food options is essential, especially for long journeys or when access to suitable food might be limited. Non-perishable items like energy bars, crackers, and nuts (if not an allergen) can be convenient options. However, it's important to consider the destination's customs regulations regarding food imports.

While planning is crucial, it's equally important to remain flexible and adaptable. Unexpected situations may arise, and it's essential to have a backup plan. Carrying a list of potential safe foods and being open to trying new allergen-free options can help in navigating unfamiliar dining environments.

Traveling with food allergies requires careful consideration and preparation. By taking the necessary precautions, individuals can enjoy their trips while managing their food allergies effectively.

Cooking at Home with Dietary Considerations

Cooking at home provides greater control over ingredients and allows for precise tailoring of meals to specific dietary needs. However, it requires careful planning, knowledge, and creativity.

Understanding Dietary Restrictions: A thorough understanding of the specific dietary requirements is essential. Researching ingredients, permitted and prohibited foods, and appropriate substitutes is crucial. Consulting with a registered dietitian or nutritionist can provide valuable guidance.

Ingredient Sourcing: Finding suitable ingredients can be challenging, especially for less common dietary restrictions. Exploring specialty grocery stores, online retailers, or farmers markets can help expand options. Building relationships with local farmers or producers can provide access to fresh, high-quality products.

Recipe Adaptation: Many traditional recipes require modifications to accommodate dietary restrictions. Experimenting with alternative ingredients and cooking techniques is essential. Online resources, cookbooks, and food blogs dedicated to specific diets can provide inspiration and guidance.

Cross-Contamination Prevention: Maintaining a clean kitchen environment is crucial to prevent cross-contamination. Using separate utensils, cutting boards, and cookware for allergen-free foods can help minimize the risk of exposure. Thoroughly washing hands, equipment, and surfaces between food preparations is essential.

Meal Planning and Preparation: Planning meals in advance can streamline the cooking process and reduce stress. Creating a weekly meal plan helps in organizing grocery lists and ensuring a variety of nutritious options. Batch cooking can save time and effort by preparing large quantities of ingredients or base dishes in advance.

Cooking at home with dietary considerations demands patience, creativity, and experimentation. With careful planning and preparation, it is possible to create delicious and satisfying meals that meet specific dietary needs.

Chapter 3 : Creating a Nutritious Diet

Building Balanced Meals with Dietary Restrictions

Constructing balanced meals while adhering to dietary restrictions requires careful planning and knowledge of nutrient sources. The goal is to ensure adequate intake of macronutrients (proteins, carbohydrates, and fats) and micronutrients (vitamins and minerals).

Understanding Nutritional Needs: Familiarizing oneself with the specific nutritional requirements of the dietary restriction is crucial. Consulting with a registered dietitian can provide personalized guidance.

Protein Sources: Identifying alternative protein sources is essential. For vegetarians and vegans, options include legumes, tofu, tempeh, lentils, quinoa, and plant-based protein powders. Individuals with dairy restrictions can explore plant-based milk alternatives fortified with calcium.

Carbohydrate Choices: Opting for whole grains, fruits, and vegetables provides a balanced intake of carbohydrates. Exploring gluten-free alternatives like quinoa, brown rice, and buckwheat can be beneficial for those following gluten-free diets.

Healthy Fats: Incorporating sources of healthy fats like avocados, nuts, seeds, and olive oil is important for overall health. However, individuals with specific dietary restrictions may need to explore alternative options.

Vitamin and Mineral Supplementation: Depending on the severity of the dietary restrictions, supplementation may be necessary to ensure adequate intake of essential vitamins and minerals. Consulting with a healthcare professional is recommended.

Meal Planning and Preparation: Creating a meal plan helps in organizing meals and ensuring a balanced intake of nutrients. Batch cooking can save time and effort, especially when dealing with multiple dietary restrictions within a household.

Building balanced meals with dietary restrictions requires creativity and experimentation. By understanding nutritional needs, exploring alternative food sources, and careful meal planning, it is possible to create delicious and nourishing meals.

Finding Alternative Sources of Nutrients

Identifying alternative nutrient sources is crucial for individuals with dietary restrictions. It involves exploring a variety of food groups and potentially incorporating supplements to ensure optimal nutritional intake.

Protein: Plant-based sources like lentils, chickpeas, tofu, tempeh, and quinoa can replace animal-based proteins. Nuts, seeds, and certain grains also offer protein content. For individuals with specific allergies, exploring less common protein sources like hemp seeds or spirulina might be necessary.

Calcium: Dairy alternatives like almond milk, soy milk, and oat milk fortified with calcium can replace dairy products. Leafy green vegetables, tofu, and fortified plant-based yogurts are also good calcium sources.

Iron: Iron-rich plant-based foods include lentils, chickpeas, spinach, fortified cereals, and tofu. Combining these foods with vitamin C-rich sources like citrus fruits can enhance iron absorption.

Vitamin B12: Primarily found in animal products, vitamin B12 deficiency is common among vegans. Fortified plant-based milk, nutritional yeast, and supplements can help meet the body's requirements.

Omega-3 Fatty Acids: Found in abundance in fatty fish, plant-based sources of omega-3 fatty acids include flaxseeds, chia seeds, walnuts, and seaweed.

Zinc: Legumes, nuts, seeds, and whole grains are good plant-based sources of zinc. However, absorption can be lower compared to animal sources.

It's essential to consult with a healthcare professional or registered dietitian to determine specific nutrient needs and to find suitable alternatives based on individual dietary restrictions.

Meal Planning and Preparation Tips

Effective meal planning and preparation can significantly simplify life, especially for individuals with dietary restrictions. It saves time, reduces food waste, and ensures a consistent intake of essential nutrients.

Start with a Plan: Begin by assessing your schedule for the week. Identify days when you have more time to cook and those when you need quick and easy options. Consider your dietary restrictions and preferences when creating a meal plan.

Create a Shopping List: Based on your meal plan, create a detailed shopping list. Grouping items by store section can streamline your grocery trip. Consider buying in bulk for staples like grains, beans, and nuts to save money.

Involve Your Pantry: Take inventory of your pantry, refrigerator, and freezer before creating a shopping list. This helps avoid unnecessary purchases and reduces food waste.

Prep Ahead: Dedicate a specific time for meal preparation. Wash and chop vegetables, cook grains, and prepare protein sources in advance. Portioning meals into individual containers can save time during busy weekdays.

Leftover Magic: Repurpose leftovers into new meals. Create soups, stews, or stir-fries using leftover cooked grains, proteins, and vegetables.

Freeze for Later: Prepare extra portions of meals and freeze them for busy days or unexpected guests. This saves time and reduces the need for last-minute meal decisions.

Keep it Simple: Don't overcomplicate your meal plans. Start with a few core recipes and gradually expand your repertoire. Focus on whole, unprocessed foods for a healthy and balanced diet.

Be Flexible: Unexpected events can disrupt meal plans. Having a few go-to quick and easy options can save the day. Don't be afraid to adapt your plan as needed.

By following these tips, you can create a meal planning routine that suits your lifestyle and dietary needs.

The Role of Supplements

Supplements can be a valuable tool in bridging nutritional gaps, especially for individuals with dietary restrictions. However, it's essential to view them as a complement to a balanced diet, not a replacement.

When to Consider Supplements:

Nutrient Deficiencies: If blood tests indicate deficiencies in specific vitamins or minerals, supplementation may be necessary.

Restricted Diets: Vegans and vegetarians may require supplements like vitamin B12 and iron.

Digestive Issues: Conditions like celiac disease or Crohn's disease can impair nutrient absorption, necessitating supplementation.

Specific Health Concerns: Certain health conditions may benefit from targeted supplementation, but consultation with a healthcare provider is crucial.

Choosing the Right Supplements:

Consult a Healthcare Professional: A doctor or registered dietitian can recommend appropriate supplements based on individual needs.

Quality Matters: Opt for reputable brands that undergo third-party testing to ensure purity and potency.

Start Low, Go Slow: Begin with lower doses and gradually increase as needed, monitoring for any side effects.

Consider Interactions: Inform your healthcare provider about all medications and supplements you're taking to avoid potential interactions.

Important Considerations:

Supplements are not regulated as strictly as medications, so their efficacy and safety can vary.

It's essential to focus on obtaining nutrients primarily through whole foods.

Excessive supplementation can lead to adverse effects.

While supplements can be beneficial in certain circumstances, they should not replace a well-balanced diet. Always consult with a healthcare professional before starting any new supplement regimen.

Addressing Common Nutritional Concerns

Navigating dietary restrictions often involves addressing common nutritional concerns. By understanding these challenges and implementing appropriate strategies, individuals can optimize their overall health and well-being.

Common Nutritional Concerns:

Nutrient Deficiencies: Restricted diets may limit the intake of essential vitamins, minerals, and macronutrients. It's crucial to monitor nutrient levels through regular blood tests and consider supplementation if necessary.

Weight Management: Balancing calorie intake with energy expenditure can be challenging, especially with certain dietary restrictions. Incorporating physical activity and mindful eating habits is essential.

Digestive Issues: Some dietary restrictions are implemented to manage digestive problems. However, other digestive concerns may arise due to dietary changes. Consulting with a healthcare provider can help identify and address these issues.

Food Allergies and Intolerances: Beyond the obvious challenges of avoiding allergens or triggers, individuals may face nutritional imbalances. Careful meal planning and potential supplementation can help mitigate these concerns.

Social and Psychological Impact: Dietary restrictions can lead to social isolation and emotional challenges. Prioritizing mental health and building a support network is crucial.

Addressing Concerns:

Educate Yourself: Learn about the specific nutritional requirements of your dietary restrictions.

Consult a Professional: A registered dietitian can provide personalized guidance and recommendations.

Prioritize Whole Foods: Focus on incorporating a variety of nutrient-dense foods into your diet.

Read Food Labels Carefully: Understanding ingredient lists is essential for making informed choices.

Experiment with New Foods: Explore different plant-based protein sources, grains, and fruits to expand your dietary repertoire.

Practice Mindful Eating: Pay attention to hunger and fullness cues to avoid overeating or undereating.

Seek Support: Connect with others who have similar dietary restrictions to share experiences and advice.

By addressing common nutritional concerns proactively, individuals with dietary restrictions can achieve optimal health and well-being.

Chapter 4 : Overcoming Challenges

Coping with Social and Emotional Aspects of Dietary Restrictions

Living with dietary restrictions can present significant social and emotional challenges. Navigating social situations, managing feelings of isolation, and maintaining positive body image are essential aspects of coping with these challenges.

Social Challenges:

Feeling Isolated: Exclusion from social events centered around food can lead to feelings of isolation.

Communication Difficulties: Effectively communicating dietary needs can be challenging, especially in unfamiliar social settings.

Food-Related Anxiety: Fear of accidental exposure to allergens or dietary restrictions can create anxiety in social situations.

Emotional Challenges:

Grief and Loss: Giving up favorite foods or missing out on shared food experiences can be emotionally difficult.

Body Image Issues: Restrictive diets can contribute to body image concerns and disordered eating behaviors.

Stress and Frustration: The constant planning and vigilance required for managing dietary restrictions can be overwhelming.

Coping Strategies:

Build a Support Network: Connect with others who have similar dietary restrictions to share experiences and support.

Communicate Effectively: Practice explaining your dietary needs clearly and concisely.

Explore Alternative Social Activities: Focus on activities that don't revolve around food, such as hobbies, outdoor adventures, or shared interests.

Practice Self-Care: Prioritize physical and mental well-being through exercise, relaxation techniques, and mindfulness.

Challenge Negative Thoughts: Replace negative self-talk with positive affirmations.

Seek Professional Help: If emotional challenges become overwhelming, consider seeking support from a therapist or counselor.

By understanding the social and emotional impact of dietary restrictions and implementing effective coping strategies, individuals can build resilience and maintain a positive outlook.

Communicating Dietary Needs Effectively

Effective communication is essential for individuals with dietary restrictions to navigate social and dining situations successfully. By clearly and concisely expressing your needs, you can increase the likelihood of finding suitable food options and avoiding misunderstandings.

Key Communication Strategies:

Be Clear and Specific: Clearly articulate your dietary restrictions, avoiding vague terms or generalizations. Use specific language to describe allergens or ingredients to avoid.

Carry Relevant Information: Having a written list of allergens or dietary needs can be helpful, especially in unfamiliar settings.

Practice Active Listening: Pay attention to the server's responses and ask clarifying questions to ensure understanding.

Be Assertive: Politely but firmly express your needs without feeling apologetic or embarrassed.

Educate Others: Take opportunities to educate friends, family, and restaurant staff about your dietary restrictions.

Utilize Technology: Many restaurants offer online menus or allergen information. Use these resources to research options in advance.

Be Patient and Flexible: Understand that not all establishments will be knowledgeable about dietary restrictions. Be prepared to offer suggestions or alternatives.

Additional Tips:

Practice communicating your dietary needs in different social settings to build confidence.

Consider using a food allergy card or app for easy reference.

Be prepared to explain the potential consequences of not accommodating your dietary needs.

By mastering effective communication, individuals with dietary restrictions can enhance their dining experiences and reduce stress associated with social interactions.

Building a Support Network

A strong support network is invaluable for individuals with dietary restrictions. Surrounding yourself with understanding and supportive people can significantly improve your overall well-being.

Identifying Potential Support:

Family and Friends: Start by reaching out to loved ones who are willing to listen and offer support.

Online Communities: Connect with others facing similar challenges through online forums, social media groups, or support groups.

Support Groups: Participate in in-person or online support groups to share experiences and gain valuable insights.

Healthcare Professionals: Build relationships with dietitians, allergists, or other healthcare providers who can offer guidance and support.

Nurturing Relationships:

Open Communication: Share your feelings, challenges, and triumphs with your support network.

Active Listening: Be present for others in your support network, offering empathy and understanding.

Mutual Support: Offer support to others in your network, fostering a sense of community.

Setting Boundaries: Establish healthy boundaries to protect your emotional well-being.

Benefits of a Strong Support Network:

Reduced Stress: Sharing your experiences with understanding individuals can alleviate stress.

Increased Confidence: Feeling supported can boost self-esteem and confidence in managing dietary restrictions.

Access to Information: Connecting with others can provide valuable information and resources.

Improved Quality of Life: A strong support network can enhance overall well-being and life satisfaction.

Building a supportive network takes time and effort, but the rewards are immeasurable. By investing in these relationships, individuals with dietary restrictions can create a strong foundation for managing their challenges and thriving.

Finding Online Resources and Communities

The internet offers a wealth of information and support for individuals with dietary restrictions. Leveraging online resources and communities can provide valuable knowledge, inspiration, and connection.

Finding Relevant Resources:

Search Engines: Utilize keywords related to your specific dietary restrictions (e.g., "gluten-free recipes," "vegan nutrition") to find websites, blogs, and articles.

Social Media: Platforms like Instagram, Facebook, and Pinterest offer a vast array of food-related content, including accounts dedicated to specific dietary restrictions.

Online Forums and Communities: Participate in online forums and communities to connect with others facing similar challenges.

Government and Health Organizations: Websites of reputable organizations often provide reliable information and resources.

Utilizing Online Communities:

Share Experiences: Connect with others who understand your challenges and share your experiences.

Seek Advice: Ask questions and get recommendations from community members.

Find Support: Build relationships with like-minded individuals for emotional support.

Discover New Resources: Learn about new products, recipes, and restaurants through community recommendations.

Important Considerations:

Evaluate Information: Not all online information is accurate. Cross-reference information from multiple sources.

Privacy Settings: Be mindful of personal information shared online.

Balance Screen Time: While online communities offer valuable support, it's essential to maintain a healthy balance between online and offline interactions.

By effectively utilizing online resources and communities, individuals with dietary restrictions can expand their knowledge, connect with others, and improve their overall well-being.

Chapter 5 : Specific Dietary Restrictions and Allergies

In-Depth Information on Specific Dietary Conditions

Understanding the specifics of a dietary condition is crucial for effective management. While this section cannot provide comprehensive medical advice, it can offer a general overview of common conditions.

Celiac Disease

Celiac disease is an autoimmune disorder triggered by the consumption of gluten, a protein found in wheat, barley, and rye. The only treatment is a strict lifelong gluten-free diet. Managing celiac disease involves carefully reading food labels, understanding hidden sources of gluten, and finding suitable gluten-free alternatives.

Diabetes

Diabetes is a chronic condition characterized by high blood sugar levels. While not strictly a dietary restriction, managing diabetes often involves careful carbohydrate intake and overall diet control. Diabetes management includes meal planning, regular blood sugar monitoring, and incorporating physical activity.

Irritable Bowel Syndrome (IBS)

IBS is a common digestive disorder characterized by symptoms like abdominal pain,bloating, and changes in bowel habits. While there's no specific diet for IBS, many people find relief by following a low-FODMAP diet. This involves limiting foods containing fermentable oligosaccharides, disaccharides, monosaccharides, and polyols.

Note: This information is intended for general knowledge and does not replace professional medical advice. Individuals with these or other dietary conditions should consult with healthcare providers for personalized guidance and treatment plans.

Common Allergies

Peanut Allergy

Peanut allergies are among the most severe and life-threatening food allergies. Individuals with peanut allergies must strictly avoid peanuts and products containing peanut traces. This includes a wide range of foods, from obvious sources like peanut butter to hidden ones like certain candies and processed foods.

Managing a peanut allergy involves meticulous label reading, inquiring about ingredients when dining out, and carrying emergency medication like epinephrine. Creating a safe home environment, educating family and friends about the severity of the allergy, and avoiding cross-contamination are essential for preventing allergic reactions.

Shellfish Allergy

Shellfish allergies encompass reactions to crustaceans (shrimp, crab, lobster) and mollusks (clams, oysters, mussels). While less common than peanut allergies, shellfish allergies can still cause severe reactions.

Individuals with shellfish allergies must carefully read food labels and inquire about ingredients when eating out. Cross-contamination is a significant concern, especially in restaurants that prepare both shellfish and non-shellfish dishes. Carrying emergency medication and informing dining companions about the allergy is crucial for managing this condition.

Note: This information is a brief overview and does not replace professional medical advice. Individuals with peanut or shellfish allergies should consult with allergists for personalized guidance and management plans.

Conclusion

take control of your dietary health

You've got this.

Every step, no matter how small, is progress. Believe in your ability to overcome challenges and reach new heights. Remember, it's not about perfection, but persistence. Keep moving forward, one day at a time.

Let's create a world where everyone feels welcome at the table.

Imagine a place where dining out isn't a stressful ordeal, but a joyful experience for everyone. That's the kind of food environment we're aiming for. It's about more than just offering gluten-free options; it's about making everyone feel valued and included.

Here's how we can make it happen:

Spread kindness and understanding: Let's educate ourselves about different dietary needs and be patient with others.

Celebrate diversity: Embrace a variety of cuisines and flavors.

Support businesses that care: Choose to dine at places that prioritize inclusivity.

Lead by example: Share your knowledge and encourage others to be mindful of dietary restrictions.

Together, we can create a food culture where everyone feels comfortable and celebrated. Let's make it happen.

The future of food is inclusive and exciting.

Imagine a world where dietary restrictions are no longer barriers to enjoying delicious, nutritious meals. That future is closer than we think. With advancements in technology, agriculture, and food science, we're on the brink of a food revolution.

Let's look ahead to what's possible:

Personalized nutrition: Tailored meal plans based on individual needs and preferences.

Allergen-free food production: Innovative methods to eliminate allergens from our food supply.

Sustainable and ethical food systems: A world where everyone has access to healthy, affordable food.

Breaking down barriers: Continued efforts to make dining out a pleasurable experience for everyone.

It's an exciting time to be part of this movement. Let's work together to shape a future where food is a source of joy and nourishment for all. Thank you.

About the Author

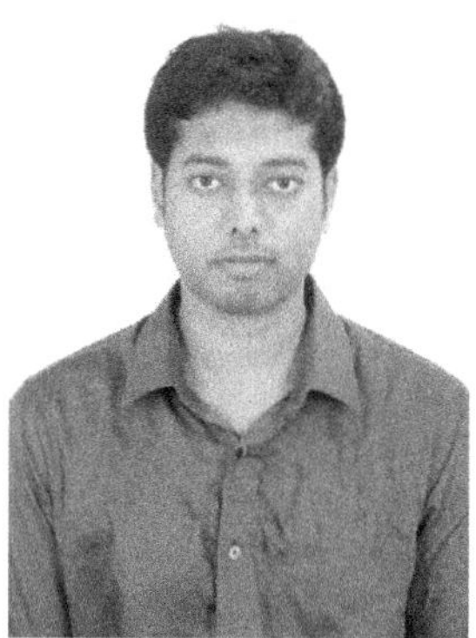

Labanya Tandi is a distinguished science fiction author based in India, celebrated for his visionary approach and narrative depth. Renowned for blending cutting-edge technology with the intricacies of human nature, Labanya crafts stories that both captivate and provoke thoughtful reflection.

From an early age, Labanya's dual passion for literature and science set the foundation for his career in speculative fiction. His Bachelor's degree in Electrical Engineering enriches his narratives with a meticulous understanding of scientific principles and technological advancements. This academic background, coupled with his dedication to rigorous research, ensures that each of his novels not only entertains but also challenges readers to contemplate the implications of future technologies.

Labanya made his literary debut with the groundbreaking work <u>**Lost in Love : Loves La*byrinth***</u>, which garnered acclaim for its innovative storytelling and exploration of futuristic themes. As a leading voice in Indian science fiction, he delves into topics such as artificial intelligence, space exploration, and the ethical dilemmas posed by technological progress. His work reflects a profound interest in the intersection of science, society, and human experience.

Residing in India, Labanya draws inspiration from the cultural richness and vibrant spirit of his surroundings. Beyond his writing, he enjoys traveling, further enriching his perspectives and experiences.

For the latest updates on Labanya's projects and to explore more about his visionary tales, visit his official website at www.labanyatandi.com.

If you've enjoyed **Dietary Restrictions and Allergies** , please consider leaving a review. Your feedback is invaluable and helps other readers discover the book. Thank You.

(The End)

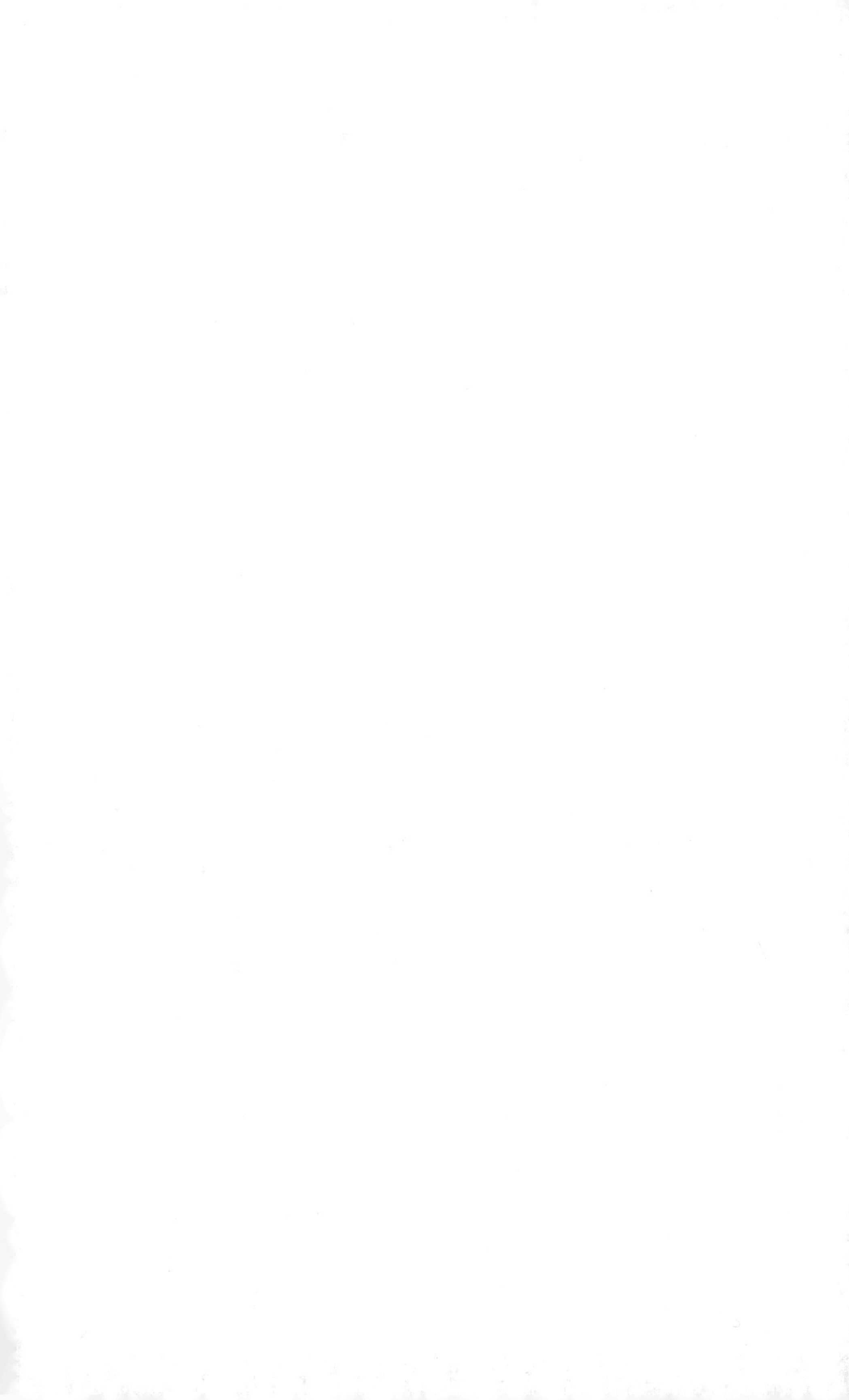

www.ingramcontent.com/pod-product-compliance
Lightning Source LLC
Chambersburg PA
CBHW051715250726
48653CB00007B/3039